I0781985

Smoothie Secrets for Weight Loss

Your Guide to Tasty and Healthy Shakes

Victor C. Sell

Copyright©2024 Victor C. Sell

All right reserved. No part of this publication may be reproduced, distributed, or transmitted in any form or by any means, including photocopying, recording, or other electronic or mechanical methods, without the prior written permission of the publisher, except in the case of brief quotation embodied in critical reviews and certain other noncommercial uses permitted by copyright law.

Table of Contents

- High-protein smoothie recipes for muscle building and fat loss

8. Fiber-Rich Smoothies
- The role of fiber in weight management
- Delicious fiber-packed smoothie recipes

9. Green Smoothies for Detox and Weight Loss
- Benefits of green smoothies
- Tasty green smoothie recipes for detox and weight loss

10. Smoothies for Meal Replacement
- Using smoothies as meal replacements
- Satisfying meal replacement smoothie recipes

11. Pre- and Post-Workout Smoothies
- Nutritional needs before and after workouts
- Energizing and recovery smoothie recipes

12. Smoothies for Breakfast
- Quick and nutritious breakfast smoothie recipes
- Tips for making smoothies part of your morning routine

13. Smoothies for Snacks and Desserts
- Healthy snack and dessert smoothie recipes
- How to satisfy sweet cravings with smoothies

14. Smoothies on a Budget
- Budget-friendly ingredients

Introduction: The Power of Smoothies

Welcome to **"Smoothie Secrets for Weight Loss: Your Guide to Tasty and Healthy Shakes."** In this book, you will discover how smoothies can be a powerful tool for achieving your weight loss goals while delighting your taste buds. Let's explore the many benefits, nutritional value, and overall health advantages that smoothies can offer.

Benefits of Smoothies for Weight Loss

Smoothies are an excellent addition to a weight loss plan for several reasons:

1. Portion Control: Smoothies allow for precise control over ingredients and portion sizes, helping you avoid overeating.
2. Nutrient Density: By blending a variety of fruits, vegetables, and other nutrient-dense ingredients, you can create a meal or snack that is packed with essential vitamins and minerals while keeping calories in check.
3. Satiety: The fiber content in fruits and vegetables helps you feel full and satisfied, reducing the likelihood of snacking on unhealthy foods.
4. Hydration: Many smoothie ingredients, like fruits and vegetables, have high water content, which aids in hydration and can support weight loss efforts.
5. Convenience: Smoothies are quick and easy to prepare, making them a convenient option for busy lifestyles. This helps you stay on track with your weight loss goals even when you're short on time.

Nutritional Value and Health Benefits

Smoothies are not only beneficial for weight loss but also contribute to overall health in several ways:

1. Vitamins and Minerals: By incorporating a variety of fruits and vegetables, smoothies provide a wide range of vitamins (such as vitamin C, A, and K) and minerals (like potassium, magnesium, and calcium) essential for maintaining good health.
2. Antioxidants: Many smoothie ingredients, such as berries, spinach, and kale, are rich in antioxidants. These compounds help protect your body from oxidative stress and inflammation, which can lead to chronic diseases.
3. Fiber: The fiber content in smoothies aids digestion, promotes gut health, and helps regulate blood sugar levels, contributing to sustained energy and reduced cravings.
4. Protein: Adding protein sources such as Greek yogurt, protein powder, or nut butters can enhance muscle repair and growth, support metabolism, and keep you fuller for longer.
5. Healthy Fats: Including sources of healthy fats, like avocado, chia seeds, or flaxseeds, can improve heart health, support brain function, and provide sustained energy.

Smoothies offer a delicious and versatile way to nourish your body while working towards your weight loss goals. With the right combination of ingredients, you can create smoothies that are not only effective for weight loss but also enhance your overall well-being. In the following chapters, you will find a variety of recipes and practical tips to help you make the most of your smoothie journey. Enjoy the journey to a healthier, happier you!

Getting Started: Essential Tools and Ingredients

Embarking on your smoothie journey begins with equipping your kitchen with the right tools and ingredients. With these essentials, you can create a wide range of delicious and nutritious weight loss smoothies.

Must-Have Kitchen Tools

1. High-Speed Blender: A powerful blender is essential for creating smooth, creamy smoothies. Look for one with multiple speed settings and strong blades to handle a variety of ingredients.

2. Measuring Cups and Spoons: Precision in measuring ingredients helps maintain portion control and ensures the right balance of nutrients.

3. Mason Jars or Reusable Bottles: These are perfect for storing and transporting your smoothies, making it easy to enjoy them on the go.

4. Cutting Board and Knife: Prepping fruits and vegetables is a breeze with a good-quality cutting board and sharp knife.

5. Ice Cube Trays: These can be used to freeze ingredients like spinach or yogurt into portioned cubes, making smoothie preparation quick and convenient.

Key Ingredients for Weight Loss Smoothies

1. Leafy Greens: Spinach, kale, and other leafy greens are low in calories and high in fiber, vitamins, and minerals.
2. Fruits: Berries, bananas, apples, and citrus fruits add natural sweetness, flavor, and essential nutrients.
3. Protein Sources: Greek yogurt, protein powder, silken tofu, and nut butters help keep you full and support muscle health.
4. Healthy Fats: Avocado, chia seeds, flaxseeds, and nuts provide sustained energy and support overall health.
5. Superfoods: Ingredients like matcha, spirulina, and cacao nibs can boost the nutritional value of your smoothies.

Recipes

1. Green Detox Smoothie

Ingredients:
- 1 cup spinach
- 1/2 cucumber, sliced
- 1 green apple, cored and chopped
- 1/2 lemon, juiced
- 1-inch piece of ginger, peeled and grated
- 1 cup coconut water
- Ice cubes (optional)

Instructions:
1. Add all ingredients to the blender.

2. Blend on high until smooth.

3. Pour into a glass and enjoy immediately.

2. Berry Protein Blast

Ingredients:

- 1 cup mixed berries (strawberries, blueberries, raspberries)
- 1/2 banana
- 1 scoop vanilla protein powder
- 1 cup unsweetened almond milk
- 1 tablespoon chia seeds

Instructions:

1. Place all ingredients in the blender.

2. Blend until creamy and smooth.

3. Serve chilled.

3. Tropical Avocado Smoothie

Ingredients:

- 1/2 avocado
- 1/2 cup pineapple chunks
- 1/2 mango, peeled and chopped
- 1 cup coconut milk
- 1 tablespoon flaxseeds

Instructions:

1. Combine all ingredients in the blender.

2. Blend until the mixture is smooth and creamy.

3. Pour into a glass and enjoy.

4. Chocolate Banana Smoothie

Ingredients:
- 1 banana
- 1 tablespoon cocoa powder
- 1 tablespoon almond butter
- 1 cup unsweetened almond milk
- 1 tablespoon flaxseeds

Instructions:
1. Add all ingredients to the blender.
2. Blend until smooth and well combined.
3. Serve immediately.

5. Citrus Ginger Smoothie

Ingredients:
- 1 orange, peeled and segmented
- 1/2 lemon, juiced
- 1 small carrot, peeled and chopped
- 1-inch piece of ginger, peeled and grated
- 1 cup water
- Ice cubes (optional)

Instructions:
1. Place all ingredients in the blender.
2. Blend on high until smooth and frothy.
3. Enjoy right away for maximum freshness.

With these essential tools and ingredients, you are well-equipped to start your smoothie-making journey. The recipes provided offer a variety of flavors and nutritional benefits to help you achieve your weight loss goals while enjoying delicious and satisfying shakes.

Understanding Macronutrients: The Role of Proteins, Fats, and Carbs in Smoothies

Achieving weight loss goals requires a well-balanced diet, and smoothies can play a crucial role in providing the necessary macronutrients—proteins, fats, and carbohydrates. Understanding how to balance these macronutrients is key to creating smoothies that support your weight loss journey while keeping you satisfied and nourished.

The Role of Proteins, Fats, and Carbs in Smoothies

1. **Proteins**: Proteins are essential for muscle repair and growth, hormone production, and overall body function. Including protein in your smoothies helps to keep you fuller for longer, reducing the likelihood of snacking between meals. Common protein sources for smoothies include Greek yogurt, protein powder, silken tofu, and nut butters.
2. **Fats**: Healthy fats are vital for brain health, hormone production, and energy. They also help absorb

fat-soluble vitamins (A, D, E, and K). Adding healthy
fats to your smoothies can make them more satisfying
and provide sustained energy. Avocado, chia seeds,
flaxseeds, and nuts are excellent sources of healthy
fats.
3. **Carbohydrates**: Carbs provide the body with energy.
    Choosing complex carbohydrates such as fruits,
    vegetables, and whole grains ensures a steady release
    of energy and prevents blood sugar spikes. These
    ingredients also add natural sweetness and essential
    nutrients to your smoothies.

Balancing Macronutrients for Optimal Weight Loss

For optimal weight loss, aim to balance your smoothies with a
good mix of proteins, fats, and carbs. A balanced smoothie
might include:
- Protein: 10-20 grams
- Fats: 5-10 grams
- Carbohydrates: 30-50 grams

This balance ensures that you receive sustained energy,
essential nutrients, and satiety, all of which support healthy
weight loss.

Recipes

1. Protein-Packed Berry Smoothie

Ingredients:

- 1 cup mixed berries (strawberries, blueberries, raspberries)
- 1/2 cup Greek yogurt
- 1 scoop vanilla protein powder
- 1 tablespoon almond butter
- 1 cup unsweetened almond milk
- 1 tablespoon chia seeds

Instructions:
1. Add all ingredients to the blender.
2. Blend on high until smooth.
3. Pour into a glass and enjoy immediately.

2. Creamy Avocado Green Smoothie

Ingredients:
- 1/2 avocado
- 1 cup spinach
- 1/2 banana
- 1/2 cup silken tofu
- 1 tablespoon flaxseeds
- 1 cup coconut water

Instructions:
1. Combine all ingredients in the blender.
2. Blend until smooth and creamy.
3. Serve chilled.

3. Tropical Protein Smoothie

Ingredients:
- 1/2 cup pineapple chunks
- 1/2 mango, peeled and chopped
- 1/2 banana
- 1 scoop protein powder
- 1 tablespoon chia seeds
- 1 cup coconut milk

Instructions:
1. Place all ingredients in the blender.
2. Blend until smooth and well combined.
3. Enjoy immediately.

4. Nutty Banana Smoothie

Ingredients:
- 1 banana
- 1 tablespoon peanut butter
- 1 tablespoon cocoa powder
- 1 scoop chocolate protein powder
- 1 cup unsweetened almond milk
- 1 tablespoon flaxseeds

Instructions:
1. Add all ingredients to the blender.
2. Blend until smooth and creamy.
3. Serve immediately.

5. Citrus Ginger Smoothie

__Ingredients__:

- 1 orange, peeled and segmented
- 1/2 lemon, juiced
- 1 small carrot, peeled and chopped
- 1-inch piece of ginger, peeled and grated
- 1 scoop vanilla protein powder
- 1 cup water
- Ice cubes (optional)

__Instructions__:

1. Place all ingredients in the blender.
2. Blend on high until smooth and frothy.
3. Enjoy right away for maximum freshness.

By understanding the role of macronutrients and how to balance them, you can create smoothies that not only taste great but also support your weight loss goals. These recipes provide a variety of flavors and nutritional benefits, helping you to stay on track while enjoying delicious and satisfying shakes.

Choosing the Right Fruits and Vegetables: Best Fruits for Weight Loss Smoothies, Nutritious Vegetables to Include

When it comes to creating smoothies for weight loss, selecting the right fruits and vegetables is crucial. These ingredients provide essential nutrients, fiber, and natural sweetness, all of which support your weight loss goals while keeping your smoothies delicious and satisfying.

Best Fruits for Weight Loss Smoothies

1. Berries: Strawberries, blueberries, raspberries, and blackberries are low in calories and high in fiber, antioxidants, and vitamins. They add natural sweetness without a lot of sugar.

2. Apples: Apples are rich in fiber and have a low glycemic index, making them great for controlling blood sugar levels.

3. Citrus Fruits: Oranges, lemons, limes, and grapefruits are packed with vitamin C and antioxidants. They add a refreshing, tangy flavor.

4. Pineapple: Pineapple is low in calories and contains bromelain, an enzyme that aids digestion.

5. Kiwi: Kiwi is a nutrient-dense fruit high in vitamin C, vitamin K, and fiber, and it adds a unique flavor to smoothies.

Nutritious Vegetables to Include

1. Spinach: Spinach is low in calories and high in vitamins A, C, and K, as well as iron and calcium. It blends well without overpowering the flavor of your smoothie.

2. Kale: Kale is a nutrient powerhouse, providing vitamins A, C, and K, as well as fiber and antioxidants.

3. Carrots: Carrots are high in beta-carotene, fiber, and vitamin K. They add a subtle sweetness and a vibrant color.

4. Cucumber: Cucumber is hydrating and low in calories. It adds a refreshing taste and helps with digestion.

5. Beets: Beets are rich in fiber, folate, and antioxidants. They provide a natural sweetness and a beautiful color.

Recipes

1. Berry Spinach Smoothie

Ingredients:
- 1 cup mixed berries (strawberries, blueberries, raspberries)
- 1 cup spinach
- 1/2 banana
- 1 cup unsweetened almond milk
- 1 tablespoon chia seeds

Instructions:
1. Add all ingredients to the blender.
2. Blend on high until smooth.
3. Pour into a glass and enjoy immediately.

2. Apple Kale Smoothie

Ingredients:
- 1 apple, cored and chopped
- 1 cup kale, stems removed
- 1/2 lemon, juiced
- 1/2 cucumber, sliced
- 1 cup coconut water

Instructions:

1. Combine all ingredients in the blender.
2. Blend until smooth and well combined.
3. Serve chilled.

3. Citrus Carrot Smoothie

Ingredients:
- 1 orange, peeled and segmented
- 1 small carrot, peeled and chopped
- 1/2 lemon, juiced
- 1/2 cup pineapple chunks
- 1 cup water
- Ice cubes (optional)

Instructions:
1. Place all ingredients in the blender.
2. Blend until smooth and frothy.
3. Enjoy right away for maximum freshness.

4. Kiwi Cucumber Smoothie

Ingredients:
- 2 kiwis, peeled and chopped
- 1/2 cucumber, sliced
- 1/2 banana
- 1 cup spinach
- 1 cup coconut milk

Instructions:
1. Add all ingredients to the blender.

2. Blend on high until smooth.
3. Pour into a glass and enjoy immediately.

5. Beet Berry Smoothie

<u>Ingredients</u>:
- 1 small beet, peeled and chopped
- 1 cup mixed berries (strawberries, blueberries, raspberries)
- 1/2 banana
- 1/2 cup Greek yogurt
- 1 cup water

<u>Instructions</u>:
1. Combine all ingredients in the blender.
2. Blend until smooth and creamy.
3. Serve chilled.

By choosing the right fruits and vegetables, you can create smoothies that are not only delicious but also packed with nutrients to support your weight loss journey. These recipes provide a variety of flavors and health benefits, ensuring you stay satisfied and energized throughout your day.

The Role of Superfoods in Smoothies: Superfoods and Their Benefits,

Incorporating Superfoods into Your Daily Smoothies

Superfoods are nutrient-rich ingredients that offer exceptional health benefits. Incorporating superfoods into your daily smoothies can boost their nutritional value, enhance your weight loss efforts, and promote overall well-being. This section explores some popular superfoods and their benefits, along with practical tips on how to include them in your smoothie recipes.

Superfoods and Their Benefits

1. Chia Seeds: Rich in omega-3 fatty acids, fiber, and protein, chia seeds help improve digestion, reduce inflammation, and provide sustained energy.

2. Flaxseeds: High in fiber, omega-3 fatty acids, and lignans, flaxseeds support heart health, improve digestion, and help balance hormones.

3. Matcha: A type of green tea powder, matcha is loaded with antioxidants, particularly catechins, which boost metabolism and enhance fat burning.

4. Spirulina: A blue-green algae, spirulina is packed with protein, vitamins, and minerals. It supports immune function, detoxification, and energy levels.

5. Cacao Nibs: Raw cacao nibs are rich in antioxidants, magnesium, and iron. They can improve mood, boost energy, and support cardiovascular health.

Incorporating Superfoods into Your Daily Smoothies

Adding superfoods to your smoothies is easy and convenient. Here are some tips to get started:Start Small: Begin by adding a small amount of superfoods to your smoothies and gradually increase the quantity as you get accustomed to the taste. Blend Well: Ensure that superfoods are well-blended to avoid any gritty texture.

Combine Flavors: Pair superfoods with complementary ingredients to enhance the overall flavor of your smoothies. Experiment: Try different combinations of superfoods and other ingredients to discover your favorite recipes.

Recipes

1. Chia Berry Blast

Ingredients:
- 1 cup mixed berries (strawberries, blueberries, raspberries)
- 1 tablespoon chia seeds
- 1/2 banana
- 1 cup unsweetened almond milk
- 1 tablespoon honey (optional)

Instructions:
1. Add all ingredients to the blender.
2. Blend on high until smooth.
3. Pour into a glass and enjoy immediately.

2. Flaxseed Tropical Smoothie

Ingredients:

- 1/2 cup pineapple chunks
- 1/2 mango, peeled and chopped
- 1 tablespoon flaxseeds
- 1/2 banana
- 1 cup coconut water

Instructions:

1. Combine all ingredients in the blender.
2. Blend until smooth and well combined.
3. Serve chilled.

3. Matcha Green Smoothie

Ingredients:

- 1 teaspoon matcha powder
- 1 cup spinach
- 1/2 avocado
- 1/2 banana
- 1 cup unsweetened almond milk

Instructions:

1. Place all ingredients in the blender.
2. Blend until smooth and creamy.
3. Enjoy immediately.

4. Spirulina Citrus Smoothie

Ingredients:

- 1 orange, peeled and segmented
- 1/2 lemon, juiced
- 1 small carrot, peeled and chopped
- 1 teaspoon spirulina powder
- 1 cup water
- Instructions:
- 1. Add all ingredients to the blender.
- 2. Blend on high until smooth and frothy.
- 3. Serve immediately.

5. Cacao Nib Banana Smoothie

Ingredients:
- 1 banana
- 1 tablespoon cacao nibs
- 1 tablespoon almond butter
- 1 cup unsweetened almond milk
- 1 tablespoon honey (optional)

Instructions:
1. Combine all ingredients in the blender.
2. Blend until smooth and creamy.
3. Pour into a glass and enjoy right away.

By incorporating superfoods into your daily smoothies, you can significantly enhance their nutritional value and support your weight loss journey. These recipes provide a variety of flavors and health benefits, helping you stay energized and nourished throughout the day.

Low-Calorie Smoothies: Recipes for Under 200-Calorie Smoothies, Tips for Reducing Calorie Content Without Sacrificing Taste

Smoothies are a great way to enjoy a delicious and nutritious meal or snack while managing your calorie intake. By choosing the right ingredients, you can create low-calorie smoothies that are satisfying and flavorful. This section provides tips for reducing calorie content and offers five tasty recipes, each under 200 calories.

Tips for Reducing Calorie Content Without Sacrificing Taste

1.**Use Low-Calorie Liquids:** Choose water, unsweetened almond milk, or coconut water instead of high-calorie liquids like fruit juice or sweetened yogurt.
2.**Limit High-Calorie Add-ins:** Be mindful of ingredients like nut butters, seeds, and high-sugar fruits. Use them sparingly or find lower-calorie alternatives.
3.**Incorporate Vegetables:** Adding vegetables like spinach, kale, and cucumber can bulk up your smoothie without adding many calories.
4.**Sweeten Naturally:** Use small amounts of low-calorie sweeteners like stevia or monk fruit, or rely on naturally sweet fruits like berries and citrus.

5. Watch Portion Sizes: Measure ingredients to control portions and keep calorie counts in check.

Recipes

1. Berry Spinach Delight

Ingredients:
- 1/2 cup strawberries (24 calories)
- 1/2 cup blueberries (42 calories)
- 1 cup spinach (7 calories)
- 1/2 banana (53 calories)
- 1 cup water (0 calories)

Instructions:
1. Add all ingredients to the blender.
2. Blend on high until smooth.
3. Pour into a glass and enjoy immediately.

Total Calories: 126

2. Citrus Cucumber Refresher

Ingredients:
- 1 orange, peeled and segmented (62 calories)
- 1/2 cucumber, sliced (8 calories)
- 1/2 lemon, juiced (6 calories)
- 1/2 cup pineapple chunks (41 calories)
- 1 cup water (0 calories)

<u>***Instructions***</u>:

1. Combine all ingredients in the blender.
2. Blend until smooth and frothy.
3. Serve chilled.

Total Calories: 117

3. Tropical Green Smoothie

<u>***Ingredients***</u>:

- 1/2 cup mango chunks (50 calories)
- 1/2 banana (53 calories)
- 1 cup spinach (7 calories)
- 1/2 cup unsweetened almond milk (15 calories)
- 1/2 cup water (0 calories)

<u>***Instructions***</u>:

1. Place all ingredients in the blender.
2. Blend until smooth and creamy.
3. Enjoy immediately.

Total Calories: 125

4. Kiwi Berry Bliss

<u>***Ingredients***</u>:

- 1 kiwi, peeled and chopped (42 calories)
- 1/2 cup raspberries (32 calories)
- 1/2 cup strawberries (24 calories)
- 1 cup water (0 calories)

Instructions:
1. Add all ingredients to the blender.
2. Blend until smooth.
3. Pour into a glass and enjoy right away.

Total Calories: 98

5. Carrot Ginger Zing

Ingredients:
- 1 small carrot, peeled and chopped (25 calories)
- 1/2 orange, peeled and segmented (31 calories)
- 1/2 apple, cored and chopped (47 calories)
- 1/2 inch ginger, peeled and grated (2 calories)
- 1 cup water (0 calories)

Instructions:
1. Combine all ingredients in the blender.
2. Blend on high until smooth.
3. Serve immediately.

Total Calories: 105

By following these tips and using the recipes provided, you can enjoy delicious, low-calorie smoothies that support your weight loss goals without sacrificing taste. These recipes are perfect for keeping your calorie intake in check while providing essential nutrients and satisfying your taste buds.

High-Protein Smoothies: Importance of Protein for Weight Loss, High-Protein Smoothie Recipes for Muscle Building and Fat Loss

Protein is a crucial macronutrient that plays a significant role in weight loss, muscle building, and overall health. High-protein smoothies are an excellent way to increase your protein intake while enjoying a delicious and convenient meal or snack. This section highlights the importance of protein for weight loss and provides five high-protein smoothie recipes designed to help you build muscle and lose fat.

Importance of Protein for Weight Loss

1.Promotes Satiety: Protein helps you feel fuller for longer, reducing the likelihood of overeating and snacking between meals.

2. Supports Muscle Maintenance: Adequate protein intake is essential for maintaining and building lean muscle mass, which boosts your metabolism and aids in fat loss.

3. Thermogenic Effect: Protein has a higher thermogenic effect compared to fats and carbohydrates, meaning your body burns more calories digesting protein.

4. Regulates Blood Sugar: Protein helps stabilize blood sugar levels, preventing energy crashes and sugar cravings.

High-Protein Smoothie Recipes

1. Peanut Butter Banana Protein Smoothie

Ingredients:

- 1 banana
- 1 scoop vanilla protein powder (approximately 20 grams of protein)
- 1 tablespoon peanut butter
- 1 cup unsweetened almond milk
- 1 tablespoon chia seeds

Instructions:

1. Add all ingredients to the blender.
2. Blend on high until smooth.
3. Pour into a glass and enjoy immediately.

Total Protein: Approximately 25 grams

2. Chocolate Avocado Protein Smoothie

Ingredients:

- 1/2 avocado
- 1 scoop chocolate protein powder (approximately 20 grams of protein)
- 1 tablespoon cocoa powder
- 1/2 banana
- 1 cup unsweetened almond milk
- 1 tablespoon flaxseeds

Instructions:

1. Combine all ingredients in the blender.
2. Blend until smooth and creamy.
3. Serve chilled.

Total Protein: Approximately 24 grams

3. Berry Greek Yogurt Protein Smoothie

Ingredients:
- 1 cup mixed berries (strawberries, blueberries, raspberries)
- 1/2 cup Greek yogurt (approximately 10 grams of protein)
- 1 scoop vanilla protein powder (approximately 20 grams of protein)
- 1 tablespoon almond butter
- 1 cup water

Instructions:
1. Place all ingredients in the blender.
2. Blend until smooth and well combined.
3. Enjoy immediately.

Total Protein: Approximately 30 grams

4. Tropical Tofu Protein Smoothie

Ingredients:
- 1/2 cup pineapple chunks
- 1/2 mango, peeled and chopped

- 1/2 cup silken tofu (approximately 10 grams of protein)
- 1 scoop vanilla protein powder (approximately 20 grams of protein)
- 1 cup coconut water

Instructions:

1. Add all ingredients to the blender.
2. Blend until smooth and creamy.
3. Pour into a glass and enjoy right away.

Total Protein: Approximately 30 grams

5. Green Protein Power Smoothie

Ingredients:

- 1 cup spinach
- 1/2 avocado
- 1/2 banana
- 1 scoop vanilla protein powder (approximately 20 grams of protein)
- 1 cup unsweetened almond milk
- 1 tablespoon chia seeds

Instructions:

1. Combine all ingredients in the blender.
2. Blend on high until smooth.
3. Serve immediately.

Total Protein: Approximately 24 grams

By incorporating high-protein smoothies into your diet, you can effectively support your weight loss and muscle-building goals. These recipes provide a variety of flavors and nutritional benefits, helping you stay satisfied and energized throughout your day.

Fiber-Rich Smoothies: The Role of Fiber in Weight Management, Delicious Fiber-Packed Smoothie Recipes

Fiber is an essential nutrient that plays a significant role in weight management by promoting satiety, regulating blood sugar levels, and supporting digestive health. Including fiber-rich ingredients in your smoothies can help you feel fuller for longer and support your overall weight loss goals. This section explores the importance of fiber and offers five delicious smoothie recipes packed with fiber to help you stay healthy and satisfied.

The Role of Fiber in Weight Management

1.Promotes Satiety: Fiber-rich foods help you feel full and satisfied, reducing the tendency to overeat or snack between meals.

2.Regulates Blood Sugar: Fiber slows the absorption of sugar into the bloodstream, preventing spikes and crashes in blood sugar levels.

3.Digestive Health: Fiber adds bulk to stool, promoting regular bowel movements and preventing constipation.

4.Aids in Weight Loss: By increasing feelings of fullness and reducing calorie intake, fiber can contribute to weight loss efforts.

Delicious Fiber-Packed Smoothie Recipes

1. Berry Oatmeal Fiber Smoothie

Ingredients:
- 1/2 cup mixed berries (strawberries, blueberries, raspberries)
- 1/4 cup rolled oats (fiber-rich)
- 1/2 banana
- 1 tablespoon chia seeds
- 1 cup unsweetened almond milk

Instructions:
1. Add rolled oats and almond milk to the blender. Let them sit for 5 minutes to soften.
2. Add remaining ingredients to the blender.
3. Blend on high until smooth and creamy.
4. Pour into a glass and enjoy immediately.

2. Green Apple Spinach Fiber Smoothie

Ingredients:
- 1 green apple, cored and chopped
- 1 cup spinach
- 1/2 avocado
- 1 tablespoon flaxseeds
- 1 cup coconut water

Instructions:
1. Combine all ingredients in the blender.
2. Blend until smooth and well combined.
3. Serve chilled.

3. Pumpkin Seed Protein Fiber Smoothie

Ingredients:
- 1/4 cup pumpkin seeds (pepitas), soaked overnight for better blending
- 1 cup mixed berries (strawberries, blueberries, raspberries)
- 1/2 banana
- 1 tablespoon almond butter
- 1 cup unsweetened almond milk

Instructions:
1. Drain and rinse soaked pumpkin seeds.
2. Add all ingredients to the blender.
3. Blend on high until smooth and creamy.
4. Pour into a glass and enjoy immediately.

4. Mango Chia Fiber Smoothie

Ingredients:

- 1/2 cup mango chunks
- 1 tablespoon chia seeds
- 1/2 cup Greek yogurt
- 1/2 banana
- 1 cup water

Instructions:

1. Add all ingredients to the blender.
2. Blend until smooth and creamy.
3. Serve chilled.

5. Blueberry Flaxseed Fiber Smoothie

Ingredients:

- 1 cup blueberries
- 1 tablespoon flaxseeds
- 1/2 cup Greek yogurt
- 1/2 cup spinach
- 1 cup unsweetened almond milk

Instruction:

1. Combine all ingredients in the blender.
2. Blend until smooth and well combined.
3. Pour into a glass and enjoy immediately.

By incorporating these fiber-packed smoothies into your diet, you can increase your fiber intake and support your weight loss and overall health goals. These recipes offer a variety of flavors and nutritional benefits, ensuring you stay satisfied and nourished throughout your day.

Green Smoothies for Detox and Weight Loss: Benefits of Green Smoothies, Tasty Green Smoothie Recipes for Detox and Weight Loss

Green smoothies are renowned for their detoxifying properties and their ability to support weight loss. Packed with vitamins, minerals, antioxidants, and fiber, these smoothies help cleanse the body, boost metabolism, and promote overall health. This section explores the benefits of green smoothies and offers five delicious recipes designed to aid detoxification and support your weight loss journey.

Benefits of Green Smoothies

1.Nutrient-Rich: Green leafy vegetables like spinach, kale, and parsley are rich in vitamins A, C, and K, as well as folate and minerals like iron and calcium.

2.Detoxification: Ingredients like celery, cucumber, and lemon help flush out toxins from the body and support liver function.

3.Hydration: Many green smoothie ingredients, such as cucumber and coconut water, are hydrating and support overall hydration levels.

4. Weight Loss Support: Green smoothies are low in calories and high in fiber, promoting feelings of fullness and aiding in weight management.

5. Antioxidant Boost: Ingredients like spinach and berries provide antioxidants that help combat oxidative stress and inflammation.

Tasty Green Smoothie Recipes for Detox and Weight Loss

1. Classic Green Detox Smoothie

Ingredients:
- 1 cup spinach
- 1/2 cucumber, sliced
- 1/2 green apple, cored and chopped
- 1/2 lemon, juiced
- 1 tablespoon fresh parsley
- 1 cup coconut water
- Ice cubes (optional)

Instructions:
1. Combine all ingredients in the blender.
2. Blend until smooth and well combined.

3. Add ice cubes if desired and blend again until smooth.
4. Pour into a glass and enjoy immediately.

2. Kale Pineapple Detox Smoothie

Ingredients:
- 1 cup kale, stems removed
- 1/2 cup pineapple chunks
- 1/2 banana
- 1/2 inch ginger, peeled and grated
- 1 tablespoon chia seeds
- 1 cup unsweetened almond milk

Instructions:
1. Add all ingredients to the blender.
2. Blend on high until smooth and creamy.
3. Serve chilled.

3. Spinach Avocado Detox Smoothie

Ingredients:
- 1 cup spinach
- 1/2 avocado
- 1/2 cup cucumber, sliced
- 1/2 lime, juiced
- 1 tablespoon fresh mint leaves
- 1 cup coconut water

__Instructions__:

1. Place all ingredients in the blender.
2. Blend until smooth and creamy.
3. Serve immediately.

4. Cucumber Celery Detox Smoothie

__Ingredients__:

- 1/2 cucumber, sliced
- 2 celery stalks, chopped
- 1 green apple, cored and chopped
- 1/2 lemon, juiced
- 1 tablespoon fresh parsley
- 1 cup water

__Instructions__:

1. Combine all ingredients in the blender.
2. Blend on high until smooth and well combined.
3. Pour into a glass and enjoy right away.

5. Green Tea Berry Detox Smoothie

__Ingredients__:

- 1 cup spinach
- 1/2 cup mixed berries (strawberries, blueberries, raspberries)
- 1/2 cup brewed green tea, cooled
- 1/2 banana
- 1 tablespoon honey (optional)
- Ice cubes (optional)

<u>*Instructions*</u>:
1. Add spinach, berries, and green tea to the blender.
2. Blend until smooth.
3. Add banana and honey, if using, and blend again until smooth.
4. Serve immediately over ice cubes if desired.

These green smoothie recipes are not only delicious but also packed with nutrients to support detoxification and weight loss. Incorporate them into your routine to enjoy their health benefits and refreshing flavors while achieving your wellness goals.

Smoothies for Meal Replacement: Using Smoothies as Meal Replacements, Satisfying Meal Replacement Smoothie Recipes

Smoothies can serve as convenient and nutritious meal replacements, providing essential nutrients while helping you manage your calorie intake for weight loss or maintenance. This section explores the benefits of using smoothies as meal replacements and offers five satisfying recipes designed to keep you full and energized throughout the day.

Using Smoothies as Meal Replacements

1.Convenience: Smoothies are quick and easy to prepare, making them ideal for busy mornings or as a quick lunch option.

2.Nutrient-Dense: You can pack smoothies with a variety of fruits, vegetables, protein, and healthy fats to ensure you get a balanced meal.

3. Portion Control: Smoothies can help with portion control by measuring ingredients and controlling calorie intake.

4. Satiety: Including protein, fiber, and healthy fats in your smoothies helps keep you feeling full and satisfied until your next meal.

Satisfying Meal Replacement Smoothie Recipes

1. Banana Nut Breakfast Smoothie

Ingredients:
- 1 banana
- 1/4 cup rolled oats
- 1 tablespoon almond butter
- 1 scoop vanilla protein powder
- 1 cup unsweetened almond milk
- Ice cubes (optional)

Instructions:
1. Combine all ingredients in the blender.
2. Blend until smooth and creamy.
3. Add ice cubes if desired and blend again until smooth.
4. Pour into a glass and enjoy immediately.

2. Mango Coconut Meal Replacement Smoothie

Ingredients:
- 1 cup mango chunks
- 1/2 cup Greek yogurt
- 1/4 cup coconut milk
- 1 tablespoon chia seeds
- 1 scoop vanilla protein powder
- 1 cup water

Instructions:
1. Add all ingredients to the blender.
2. Blend on high until smooth and well combined.
3. Serve chilled.

3. Spinach Berry Protein Smoothie Bowl

Ingredients:
- 1 cup spinach
- 1/2 cup mixed berries (strawberries, blueberries, raspberries)
- 1/2 banana
- 1/4 cup Greek yogurt
- 1 scoop vanilla protein powder
- Toppings: sliced almonds, chia seeds, fresh berries

Instructions:

1. Blend spinach, berries, banana, Greek yogurt, and protein powder until smooth.
2. Pour into a bowl.
3. Top with sliced almonds, chia seeds, and fresh berries.
4. Enjoy with a spoon.

4. Chocolate Almond Meal Replacement Smoothie

Ingredients:
- 1 tablespoon almond butter
- 1 tablespoon cocoa powder
- 1/2 banana
- 1 scoop chocolate protein powder
- 1 cup unsweetened almond milk
- Ice cubes (optional)

Instructions:
1. Combine all ingredients in the blender.
2. Blend until smooth and creamy.
3. Add ice cubes if desired and blend again until smooth.
4. Pour into a glass and enjoy immediately.

5. Avocado Green Tea Meal Replacement Smoothie

Ingredients:
- 1/2 avocado
- 1 cup spinach
- 1/2 cup brewed green tea, cooled
- 1/2 banana
- 1 scoop vanilla protein powder

- 1 tablespoon honey (optional)

Instructions:
1. Add avocado, spinach, green tea, banana, protein powder, and honey to the blender.
2. Blend until smooth and creamy.
3. Serve immediately.

These meal replacement smoothie recipes are nutritious, satisfying, and perfect for those looking to manage their weight or enjoy a quick, healthy meal on the go. Incorporate them into your routine to reap the benefits of balanced nutrition and convenience.

Pre- and Post-Workout Smoothies: Nutritional Needs Before and After Workouts, Energizing and Recovery Smoothie Recipes

Pre- and post-workout smoothies are essential for fueling your exercise routine, enhancing performance, and supporting muscle recovery. This section discusses the nutritional needs before and after workouts and provides five energizing and recovery smoothie recipes to optimize your fitness goals.

Nutritional Needs Before and After Workouts

1. Pre-Workout Nutrition:
- **Carbohydrates**: Provide quick energy for workouts.
- **Protein**: Supports muscle repair and growth.
- **Hydration**: Maintain fluid balance and prevent dehydration.
- **Electrolytes**: Replace electrolytes lost through sweat.

2. Post-Workout Nutrition:
- **Protein**: Essential for muscle recovery and repair.
- **Carbohydrates**: Replenish glycogen stores and aid recovery.
- **Antioxidants**: Help reduce inflammation and oxidative stress.
- **Hydration**: Replace fluids lost during exercise.

Energizing and Recovery Smoothie Recipes

1. Banana Berry Pre-Workout Smoothie

Ingredients:
- 1 banana
- 1/2 cup mixed berries (strawberries, blueberries, raspberries)
- 1/4 cup rolled oats
- 1 tablespoon honey (optional)
- 1 cup water or coconut water
- Ice cubes (optional)

<u>**Instructions**</u>:

1. Combine all ingredients in the blender.

2. Blend until smooth and creamy.

3. Add ice cubes if desired and blend again until smooth.

4. Pour into a glass and enjoy 30-60 minutes before your workout.

2. Chocolate Peanut Butter Protein Post-Workout Smoothie

<u>**Ingredients**</u>:

- 1 scoop chocolate protein powder
- 1 tablespoon peanut butter
- 1/2 banana
- 1 cup unsweetened almond milk
- Ice cubes (optional)

<u>**Instructions**</u>:

1. Add protein powder, peanut butter, banana, and almond milk to the blender.

2. Blend until smooth and creamy.

3. Add ice cubes if desired and blend again until smooth.

4. Pour into a glass and enjoy within 30 minutes after your workout.

3. Green Coconut Hydration Smoothie

<u>**Ingredients**</u>:

- 1 cup spinach
- 1/2 cup cucumber, sliced

- 1/2 cup pineapple chunks
- 1/4 cup coconut water
- Juice of 1/2 lime
- Ice cubes (optional)

Instructions:
1. Add spinach, cucumber, pineapple, coconut water, and lime juice to the blender.
2. Blend until smooth and well combined.
3. Add ice cubes if desired and blend again until smooth.
4. Pour into a glass and enjoy for hydration post-workout.

4. Blueberry Almond Recovery Smoothie

Ingredients:
- 1 cup blueberries
- 1/4 cup almonds, soaked overnight for easier blending
- 1/2 cup Greek yogurt
- 1 tablespoon honey (optional)
- 1 cup water or almond milk

Instructions:
1. Drain and rinse soaked almonds.
2. Add almonds, blueberries, Greek yogurt, honey, and water or almond milk to the blender.
3. Blend on high until smooth and creamy.
4. Pour into a glass and enjoy for muscle recovery after exercise.

5. Tropical Turmeric Anti-Inflammatory Smoothie

<u>*Ingredients*</u>:

- 1/2 cup mango chunks
- 1/2 cup pineapple chunks
- 1/2 inch fresh turmeric root, peeled and grated (or 1/2 teaspoon ground turmeric)
- 1 tablespoon chia seeds
- 1 cup coconut water
- Ice cubes (optional)

<u>*Instructions*</u>:

1. Combine mango, pineapple, turmeric, chia seeds, and coconut water in the blender.
2. Blend until smooth and well combined.
3. Add ice cubes if desired and blend again until smooth.
4. Pour into a glass and enjoy for its anti-inflammatory properties post-workout.

These pre- and post-workout smoothie recipes are designed to optimize your performance, support muscle recovery, and provide essential nutrients for overall health. Incorporate them into your fitness routine to fuel your workouts and aid recovery effectively.

Smoothies for Breakfast: Quick and Nutritious Breakfast Smoothie Recipes,

Tips for Making Smoothies Part of Your Morning Routine

Smoothies are an ideal choice for a quick and nutritious breakfast, providing a balance of essential nutrients to start your day right. This section explores the benefits of incorporating smoothies into your morning routine and offers five delicious breakfast smoothie recipes that are easy to prepare and full of flavor.

Tips for Making Smoothies Part of Your Morning Routine

1.**Prep Ingredients Ahead:** Wash and chop fruits and vegetables the night before for quicker assembly in the morning.
2.**Use Frozen Ingredients:** Frozen fruits and vegetables help create a creamy texture and eliminate the need for ice.
3.**Add Protein:** Include sources like Greek yogurt, protein powder, or nut butter to make your smoothie more satisfying and balanced.
4.**Include Fiber:** Add oats, chia seeds, or flaxseeds for added fiber to keep you full longer.
5.**Experiment with Flavors:** Blend different combinations of fruits, vegetables, and liquids to discover your favorite flavors.

Quick and Nutritious Breakfast Smoothie Recipes

1. Berry Banana Breakfast Smoothie

<u>*Ingredients*</u>:
- 1/2 cup mixed berries (strawberries, blueberries, raspberries)
- 1 banana
- 1/2 cup Greek yogurt
- 1 tablespoon honey (optional)
- 1 cup unsweetened almond milk
- Ice cubes (optional)

<u>*Instructions*</u>:
1. Combine berries, banana, Greek yogurt, honey, and almond milk in the blender.
2. Blend until smooth and creamy.
3. Add ice cubes if desired and blend again until smooth.
4. Pour into a glass and enjoy immediately.

2. Green Power Breakfast Smoothie

<u>*Ingredients*</u>:
- 1 cup spinach
- 1/2 cucumber, sliced
- 1/2 avocado
- Juice of 1/2 lime
- 1 tablespoon chia seeds
- 1 cup coconut water

<u>*Instructions*</u>:
1. Add spinach, cucumber, avocado, lime juice, chia seeds, and coconut water to the blender.
2. Blend until smooth and well combined.

3. Serve chilled.

3. Peanut Butter Banana Protein Smoothie

Ingredients:
- 1 banana
- 1 tablespoon peanut butter
- 1 scoop vanilla protein powder
- 1/4 cup rolled oats
- 1 cup unsweetened almond milk
- Ice cubes (optional)

Instructions:
1. Combine banana, peanut butter, protein powder, rolled oats, and almond milk in the blender.
2. Blend until smooth and creamy.
3. Add ice cubes if desired and blend again until smooth.
4. Pour into a glass and enjoy immediately.

4. Mango Coconut Chia Smoothie Bowl

Ingredients:
- 1 cup mango chunks
- 1/2 cup Greek yogurt
- 1/4 cup coconut milk
- 1 tablespoon chia seeds
- Toppings: sliced almonds, shredded coconut, fresh berries

Instruction:

1. Blend mango, Greek yogurt, coconut milk, and chia seeds
until smooth.
2. Pour into a bowl.
3. Top with sliced almonds, shredded coconut, and fresh
berries.
4. Enjoy with a spoon.

5. Chocolate Almond Breakfast Smoothie

Ingredients:
- 1 scoop chocolate protein powder
- 1 tablespoon almond butter
- 1/2 banana
- 1 tablespoon cocoa powder
- 1 cup unsweetened almond milk
- Ice cubes (optional)

Instructions:
1. Combine protein powder, almond butter, banana, cocoa
powder, and almond milk in the blender.
2. Blend until smooth and creamy.
3. Add ice cubes if desired and blend again until smooth.
4. Pour into a glass and enjoy immediately.

These breakfast smoothie recipes are nutritious, delicious, and
perfect for busy mornings. By incorporating these recipes into
your morning routine, you can enjoy a satisfying breakfast
that fuels your day with essential nutrients and energy.

Smoothies for Snacks and Desserts: Healthy Snack and Dessert Smoothie Recipes, How to Satisfy Sweet Cravings with Smoothies

Smoothies can be a delightful choice for satisfying sweet cravings while still providing nutritious ingredients. This section explores how smoothies can serve as healthy snacks and desserts and offers five delicious recipes that are both satisfying and guilt-free.

How to Satisfy Sweet Cravings with Smoothies

1. Choose Natural Sweeteners: Use fruits like bananas, berries, or dates to add sweetness without refined sugars.
2. Include Healthy Fats: Nut butters, avocado, or coconut milk can add creaminess and satiety to dessert smoothies.
3. Experiment with Flavors: Blend different combinations of fruits, vegetables, and spices to create unique and satisfying flavors.
4. Add Protein: Include protein powder or Greek yogurt to make your smoothie more filling and balanced.
5. Enjoy in Moderation: While nutritious, smoothies can still be calorie-dense, so enjoy them as part of a balanced diet.

Healthy Snack and Dessert Smoothie Recipes

1. Peanut Butter Banana Smoothie

Ingredients:
- 1 banana
- 1 tablespoon peanut butter
- 1/2 cup Greek yogurt
- 1 tablespoon honey (optional)
- 1 cup unsweetened almond milk
- Ice cubes (optional)

Instructions:
1. Combine banana, peanut butter, Greek yogurt, honey, and almond milk in the blender.
2. Blend until smooth and creamy.
3. Add ice cubes if desired and blend again until smooth.
4. Pour into a glass and enjoy as a satisfying snack or dessert.

2. Chocolate Avocado Smoothie Bowl

Ingredients:
- 1/2 avocado
- 1 tablespoon cocoa powder
- 1 tablespoon honey or maple syrup
- 1/2 cup Greek yogurt
- 1/2 cup unsweetened almond milk
- Toppings: sliced almonds, dark chocolate shavings, fresh berries

<u>*Instructions*</u>:

1. Blend avocado, cocoa powder, honey or maple syrup, Greek yogurt, and almond milk until smooth.
2. Pour into a bowl.
3. Top with sliced almonds, dark chocolate shavings, and fresh berries.
4. Enjoy with a spoon as a nutritious dessert option.

3. Berry Almond Smoothie

<u>*Ingredients*</u>:

- 1 cup mixed berries (strawberries, blueberries, raspberries)
- 1/4 cup almonds, soaked overnight for easier blending
- 1/2 cup Greek yogurt
- 1 tablespoon honey (optional)
- 1 cup water or almond milk

<u>*Instructions*</u>:

1. Drain and rinse soaked almonds.
2. Combine berries, almonds, Greek yogurt, honey, and water or almond milk in the blender.
3. Blend on high until smooth and creamy.
4. Pour into a glass and enjoy as a refreshing and nutritious snack.

4. Mango Coconut Chia Dessert Smoothie

<u>*Ingredients*</u>:

- 1 cup mango chunks

- 1/4 cup coconut milk
- 1 tablespoon chia seeds
- 1/2 cup Greek yogurt
- 1 tablespoon honey or maple syrup
- Ice cubes (optional)

Instructions:

1. Blend mango, coconut milk, chia seeds, Greek yogurt, and honey or maple syrup until smooth.
2. Add ice cubes if desired and blend again until smooth.
3. Pour into a glass.
4. Enjoy as a creamy and satisfying dessert alternative.

5. Green Tea Berry Smoothie

Ingredients:

- 1 cup mixed berries (strawberries, blueberries, raspberries)
- 1/2 cup brewed green tea, cooled
- 1/2 cup Greek yogurt
- 1 tablespoon honey or maple syrup
- Ice cubes (optional)

Instructions:

1. Blend berries, green tea, Greek yogurt, and honey or maple syrup until smooth.
2. Add ice cubes if desired and blend again until smooth.
3. Pour into a glass.

4. Enjoy as a refreshing and antioxidant-rich snack or dessert option.

These smoothie recipes are perfect for satisfying sweet cravings while providing essential nutrients. Whether enjoyed as a snack or dessert, these options are delicious, nutritious, and support your overall wellness goals.

Smoothies on a Budget: Budget-Friendly Ingredients, Cost-Effective Smoothie Recipes

Smoothies can be both nutritious and budget-friendly by using simple ingredients that are readily available and affordable. This section focuses on cost-effective smoothie recipes that prioritize economical ingredients without compromising on taste or health benefits.

Budget-Friendly Ingredients for Smoothies

1. Frozen Fruits: Often more affordable than fresh fruits and provide a longer shelf life.
2. Leafy Greens: Spinach and kale are nutritious and cost-effective choices for adding greens to smoothies.
3. Oats: Rolled oats add fiber and bulk to smoothies at a low cost.

4. Bananas: A versatile fruit that adds sweetness and creaminess to smoothies.

5. Greek Yogurt: Provides protein and creaminess, often available in larger, cost-effective containers.

6. Nut Butters: Adds flavor, healthy fats, and protein to smoothies in small quantities.

7. Milk Alternatives: Almond milk, soy milk, or oat milk can be cost-effective options compared to dairy milk.

Cost-Effective Smoothie Recipes

1. Berry Oatmeal Smoothie

Ingredients:
- 1/2 cup mixed berries (strawberries, blueberries, raspberries)
- 1/4 cup rolled oats
- 1/2 banana
- 1/2 cup Greek yogurt
- 1 tablespoon honey (optional)
- 1 cup water or milk of choice

Instructions:
1. Combine mixed berries, rolled oats, banana, Greek yogurt, honey, and water or milk in the blender.
2. Blend until smooth and creamy.
3. Pour into a glass and enjoy as a nutritious and filling smoothie.

2. Green Banana Smoothie

Ingredients:
- 1 banana
- 1 cup spinach
- 1/2 cup Greek yogurt
- 1 tablespoon peanut butter
- 1 tablespoon honey (optional)
- 1 cup water or milk of choice

Instructions:
1. Blend banana, spinach, Greek yogurt, peanut butter, honey, and water or milk until smooth.
2. Pour into a glass and serve immediately.

3. Tropical Mango Smoothie

Ingredients:
- 1 cup frozen mango chunks
- 1/2 cup pineapple chunks (fresh or canned in juice)
- 1/2 banana
- 1/2 cup coconut water or water
- Juice of 1/2 lime

Instruction:
1. Blend mango, pineapple, banana, coconut water or water, and lime juice until smooth.
2. Pour into a glass and enjoy this refreshing tropical smoothie.

4. Chocolate Peanut Butter Banana Smoothie

Ingredients:
- 1 banana
- 1 tablespoon cocoa powder
- 1 tablespoon peanut butter
- 1/2 cup Greek yogurt
- 1 tablespoon honey or maple syrup (optional)
- 1 cup almond milk or milk of choice

Instructions:
1. Blend banana, cocoa powder, peanut butter, Greek yogurt, honey or maple syrup, and almond milk until smooth.
2. Pour into a glass and enjoy this indulgent yet budget-friendly smoothie.

5. Berry Spinach Smoothie

Ingredients:
- 1 cup spinach
- 1/2 cup mixed berries (strawberries, blueberries, raspberries)
- 1/2 banana
- 1/2 cup Greek yogurt
- 1 tablespoon honey (optional)
- 1 cup water or milk of choice

Instructions:

1. Blend spinach, mixed berries, banana, Greek yogurt, honey, and water or milk until smooth.
2. Pour into a glass and savor the nutritional benefits of this simple and cost-effective smoothie.

These budget-friendly smoothie recipes are perfect for those looking to enjoy nutritious and delicious beverages without breaking the bank. Incorporate these recipes into your routine to support your health goals while staying mindful of your budget.

Smoothies for Special Dietary Needs: Vegan, Gluten-Free, and Dairy-Free Options, Recipes Catering to Various Dietary Restrictions

Smoothies can be adapted to accommodate various dietary needs, including vegan, gluten-free, and dairy-free preferences. This section explores recipes that cater to these dietary restrictions while ensuring they remain tasty, nutritious, and suitable for weight loss goals.

Tips for Special Dietary Needs

1. Substitute Dairy: Use plant-based milk alternatives such as almond milk, soy milk, or oat milk instead of dairy milk.

2. Replace Yogurt: Opt for dairy-free yogurt made from coconut, almond, or soy for creamy texture and probiotic benefits.

3. Gluten-Free Grains: Choose gluten-free grains like rolled oats or quinoa flakes to add fiber and texture to smoothies.

4. Natural Sweeteners: Use honey, maple syrup, or dates as sweeteners instead of refined sugars for added health benefits.

Recipes Catering to Various Dietary Restrictions

1. Vegan Berry Spinach Smoothie

Ingredients:
- 1 cup spinach
- 1/2 cup mixed berries (strawberries, blueberries, raspberries)
- 1/2 banana
- 1 tablespoon chia seeds
- 1 cup almond milk or coconut water

Instructions:
1. Blend spinach, mixed berries, banana, chia seeds, and almond milk or coconut water until smooth.
2. Pour into a glass and enjoy this vegan-friendly and nutrient-packed smoothie.

2. Gluten-Free Mango Coconut Smoothie

Ingredients:
- 1 cup frozen mango chunks

- 1/2 cup coconut milk
- 1/2 banana
- Juice of 1/2 lime
- Ice cubes (optional)

Instructions:

1. Blend mango chunks, coconut milk, banana, and lime juice until smooth.
2. Add ice cubes if desired and blend again until smooth.
3. Pour into a glass and savor this refreshing gluten-free smoothie option.

3. Dairy-Free Green Tea Berry Smoothie

Ingredients:

- 1 cup mixed berries (strawberries, blueberries, raspberries)
- 1/2 cup brewed green tea, cooled
- 1/2 cup dairy-free yogurt (coconut or almond)
- 1 tablespoon honey or maple syrup (optional)
- Ice cubes (optional)

Instructions:

1. Blend mixed berries, green tea, dairy-free yogurt, and honey or maple syrup until smooth.
2. Add ice cubes if desired and blend again until smooth.
3. Pour into a glass and enjoy this dairy-free and antioxidant-rich smoothie.

4. Avocado Banana Chia Seed Smoothie (Vegan and Gluten-Free)

<u>*Ingredients*</u>:
- 1/2 avocado
- 1 banana
- 1 tablespoon chia seeds
- 1 tablespoon honey or agave syrup (optional)
- 1 cup almond milk or coconut water

<u>*Instructions*</u>:
1. Blend avocado, banana, chia seeds, honey or agave syrup, and almond milk or coconut water until smooth.
2. Pour into a glass and indulge in this creamy and nutrient-dense vegan and gluten-free smoothie.

5. Pineapple Ginger Turmeric Smoothie (Vegan and Dairy-Free)

<u>*Ingredients*</u>:
- 1 cup pineapple chunks
- 1/2 inch fresh ginger, peeled
- 1/2 teaspoon ground turmeric
- 1 tablespoon chia seeds
- 1 cup coconut water or almond milk

<u>*Instructions*</u>:
1. Blend pineapple chunks, ginger, turmeric, chia seeds, and coconut water or almond milk until smooth.

2. Pour into a glass and enjoy this vibrant and immune-boosting vegan and dairy-free smoothie option.

These smoothie recipes cater to various dietary restrictions, ensuring everyone can enjoy delicious and nutritious beverages that support their health and weight loss goals. Incorporate these recipes into your routine to explore new flavors while accommodating your dietary preferences.

Smoothies for Busy Lifestyles: Quick and Easy Smoothie Recipes, Tips for Preparing Smoothies in Advance

Smoothies are perfect for those with hectic schedules, providing a quick and nutritious option that can be prepared in minutes. This section focuses on easy-to-make smoothie recipes and tips for preparing them ahead of time to fit seamlessly into busy lifestyles.

Tips for Preparing Smoothies in Advance

1. Prep Smoothie Packs: Pre-measure and pack smoothie ingredients in freezer-safe bags or containers for quick blending.

2. Freeze Ingredients: Freeze fruits like bananas, berries, and spinach to maintain freshness and texture.

3. Use Frozen Ingredients: Frozen fruits eliminate the need for ice and help create a thicker, creamier smoothie.

4. Store in Mason Jars: Prepare smoothies in advance and store them in sealed mason jars in the refrigerator for grab-and-go convenience.

5. Batch Preparation: Make larger batches of smoothies and store them in individual servings in the freezer for longer-term storage.

Quick and Easy Smoothie Recipes

1. Banana Almond Butter Smoothie

Ingredients:
- 1 banana, frozen
- 1 tablespoon almond butter
- 1/2 cup Greek yogurt
- 1 tablespoon honey (optional)
- 1 cup almond milk or milk of choice

Instructions:
1. Place frozen banana, almond butter, Greek yogurt, honey, and almond milk in the blender.
2. Blend until smooth and creamy.
3. Pour into a glass and enjoy this protein-packed smoothie.

2. Mixed Berry Spinach Smoothie

<u>*Ingredients*</u>:

- 1 cup mixed berries (strawberries, blueberries, raspberries), frozen
- 1 cup spinach
- 1/2 cup Greek yogurt
- 1 tablespoon chia seeds
- 1 cup water or coconut water

<u>*Instructions*</u>:

1. Combine mixed berries, spinach, Greek yogurt, chia seeds, and water or coconut water in the blender.
2. Blend until smooth and well combined.
3. Pour into a glass and savor this antioxidant-rich smoothie.

3. Pineapple Coconut Green Smoothie

<u>*Ingredients*</u>:

- 1 cup pineapple chunks, frozen
- 1 cup spinach or kale
- 1/2 cup coconut milk
- Juice of 1/2 lime
- Ice cubes (optional)

<u>*Instructions*</u>:

1. Blend pineapple chunks, spinach or kale, coconut milk, and lime juice until smooth.
2. Add ice cubes if desired and blend again until smooth.

3. Pour into a glass and enjoy this tropical-inspired green smoothie.

4. Chocolate Banana Protein Smoothie

Ingredients:
- 1 banana, frozen
- 1 scoop chocolate protein powder
- 1 tablespoon cocoa powder
- 1 tablespoon almond butter
- 1 cup almond milk or milk of choice

Instructions:
1. Blend frozen banana, chocolate protein powder, cocoa powder, almond butter, and almond milk until smooth.
2. Pour into a glass and indulge in this chocolatey protein-packed smoothie.

5. Mango Turmeric Smoothie

Ingredients:
- 1 cup frozen mango chunks
- 1/2 inch fresh ginger, peeled
- 1/2 teaspoon ground turmeric
- 1 tablespoon honey or maple syrup (optional)
- 1 cup coconut water or water

Instructions:

1. Blend frozen mango chunks, fresh ginger, ground turmeric, honey or maple syrup, and coconut water or water until smooth.
2. Pour into a glass and enjoy this vibrant and immune-boosting smoothie.

These quick and easy smoothie recipes are perfect for busy lifestyles, providing nutritious options that can be prepared in advance or whipped up in minutes. Incorporate these recipes into your routine to stay energized and nourished throughout your day.

Storing and Freezing Smoothies: Proper Storage Techniques, How to Freeze and Thaw Smoothies for Later Use

Smoothies can be conveniently stored and frozen for later consumption, making them an ideal option for meal prep and busy schedules. This section covers proper storage techniques and guidelines for freezing and thawing smoothies, along with five recipes that are suitable for freezing.

Proper Storage Techniques

1. Refrigeration: Store prepared smoothies in airtight containers, such as mason jars or reusable bottles, in the refrigerator for up to 2 days.

2. Freezing: Freeze smoothies in individual portions using freezer-safe containers or resealable bags for up to 3 months.

3. Avoiding Separation: If using ingredients prone to separation (like dairy or non-dairy milk), shake or stir well before consuming.

4. Thawing: Thaw frozen smoothies in the refrigerator overnight or at room temperature for a few hours. You can also thaw by placing the sealed container in a bowl of lukewarm water for quicker thawing.

5. Blending After Thawing: Blend thawed smoothies again briefly to restore consistency and texture before serving.

How to Freeze and Thaw Smoothies

1. Prepare Smoothie: Blend your desired smoothie recipe until smooth and well combined.

2. Portion: Pour the blended smoothie into individual servings or into ice cube trays for easy portioning later.

3. Freeze: Place the containers or trays in the freezer and freeze until solid.

4. Storage: Transfer frozen smoothie portions into freezer-safe bags or containers, ensuring to remove as much air as possible to prevent freezer burn.

5. Thaw: When ready to enjoy, remove the desired number of smoothie portions from the freezer and thaw using one of the methods mentioned above.

Frozen Smoothie Recipes

1. Mixed Berry Oatmeal Smoothie

Ingredients:
- 1/2 cup mixed berries (strawberries, blueberries, raspberries)
- 1/4 cup rolled oats
- 1/2 banana
- 1/2 cup Greek yogurt
- 1 tablespoon honey (optional)
- 1 cup almond milk or milk of choice

Instructions:
1. Blend mixed berries, rolled oats, banana, Greek yogurt, honey, and almond milk until smooth.
2. Pour into individual freezer-safe containers or ice cube trays.
3. Freeze until solid.
4. Thaw in the refrigerator overnight or blend frozen cubes with almond milk for a quick smoothie.

2. Green Mango Kale Smoothie

Ingredients:
- 1 cup frozen mango chunks

- 1 cup kale leaves, stems removed
- 1/2 banana
- Juice of 1/2 lime
- 1 tablespoon chia seeds
- 1 cup coconut water or water

Instructions:
1. Blend mango chunks, kale leaves, banana, lime juice, chia seeds, and coconut water or water until smooth.
2. Portion into freezer-safe containers.
3. Freeze and thaw as needed for a refreshing green smoothie.

3. Chocolate Peanut Butter Protein Smoothie

Ingredients:
- 1 banana, frozen
- 1 scoop chocolate protein powder
- 1 tablespoon peanut butter
- 1 tablespoon cocoa powder
- 1 cup almond milk or milk of choice

Instructions:
1. Blend frozen banana, chocolate protein powder, peanut butter, cocoa powder, and almond milk until smooth.
2. Divide into individual servings in freezer-safe containers.
3. Freeze and thaw overnight in the refrigerator or blend frozen with almond milk for a creamy chocolatey treat.

4. Pineapple Coconut Ginger Smoothie

<u>*Ingredients*</u>:
- 1 cup frozen pineapple chunks
- 1/2 cup coconut milk
- 1/2 inch fresh ginger, peeled
- 1 tablespoon honey or maple syrup (optional)
- 1 cup coconut water or water

<u>*Instructions*</u>:
1. Blend pineapple chunks, coconut milk, ginger, honey or maple syrup, and coconut water or water until smooth.
2. Portion into freezer-safe containers.
3. Freeze and thaw for a tropical-inspired smoothie.

5. Blueberry Spinach Avocado Smoothie

<u>*Ingredients*</u>:
- 1 cup frozen blueberries
- 1 cup spinach
- 1/2 avocado
- 1 tablespoon chia seeds
- Juice of 1/2 lemon
- 1 cup almond milk or milk of choice

<u>*Instructions*</u>:
1. Blend frozen blueberries, spinach, avocado, chia seeds, lemon juice, and almond milk until smooth.
2. Transfer into freezer-safe containers or ice cube trays.
3. Freeze and thaw overnight in the refrigerator or blend frozen cubes with almond milk for a nutritious green smoothie.

These frozen smoothie recipes are perfect for preparing ahead of time, ensuring you always have a nutritious and delicious option on hand. Follow these storage and freezing tips to maintain the quality and freshness of your smoothies for convenient consumption.

Customizing Your Smoothies: Tips for Personalizing Your Smoothie Recipes, Creative Ways to Enhance Flavor and Nutrition

Smoothies are versatile and can be customized to suit individual tastes and nutritional needs. This section explores tips for personalizing smoothie recipes and creative ways to enhance flavor and nutrition, along with five customizable recipes that cater to different preferences.

Tips for Personalizing Your Smoothie

1. Choose a Base: Start with a liquid base like almond milk, coconut water, or fruit juice for consistency.

2. Add Protein: Incorporate protein sources such as Greek yogurt, protein powder, or nut butter for satiety and muscle repair.

3. Boost with Greens: Include leafy greens like spinach, kale, or Swiss chard for added vitamins and fiber.

4. Sweeten Naturally: Use fruits like bananas, berries, or dates as natural sweeteners instead of refined sugars.

5. Enhance with Superfoods: Boost nutritional value with superfoods like chia seeds, flaxseeds, or spirulina.

6. Experiment with Flavors: Blend different fruits, vegetables, and herbs to create unique flavor combinations.

7. Adjust Texture: Add ice cubes or frozen fruits for a thicker, creamier texture.

Creative Ways to Enhance Flavor and Nutrition

- **Spices**: Add spices such as cinnamon, ginger, or turmeric for added flavor and health benefits.
- **Herbs**: Fresh herbs like mint, basil, or cilantro can impart refreshing flavors.
- **Citrus Zest:** Grate lemon or orange zest for a burst of citrusy flavor.

- **Coconut**: Use coconut milk, shredded coconut, or coconut water to add a tropical twist.
- **Vanilla Extract**: A dash of vanilla extract can enhance sweetness without adding sugar.

Customizable Smoothie Recipes

1. Berry-Banana Protein Smoothie

Ingredients:
- 1/2 cup mixed berries (strawberries, blueberries, raspberries)
- 1 banana
- 1 scoop vanilla protein powder
- 1 tablespoon almond butter
- 1 cup almond milk or milk of choice
- Ice cubes (optional)

Instructions:
1. Blend mixed berries, banana, vanilla protein powder, almond butter, and almond milk until smooth.
2. Add ice cubes if desired and blend again until creamy.
3. Pour into a glass and enjoy this protein-packed smoothie.

2. Tropical Green Smoothie

Ingredients:
- 1 cup spinach
- 1/2 cup frozen mango chunks
- 1/2 cup frozen pineapple chunks

- 1/2 banana
- Juice of 1/2 lime
- 1 cup coconut water or water

Instructions:

1. Blend spinach, mango chunks, pineapple chunks, banana, lime juice, and coconut water or water until smooth.
2. Adjust consistency with more liquid if needed.
3. Pour into a glass and savor this refreshing tropical green smoothie.

3. Avocado Blueberry Superfood Smoothie

Ingredients:

- 1/2 avocado
- 1 cup frozen blueberries
- 1 tablespoon chia seeds
- 1 tablespoon honey or maple syrup (optional)
- 1 cup almond milk or milk of choice

Instructions:

1. Blend avocado, frozen blueberries, chia seeds, honey or maple syrup, and almond milk until smooth.
2. Taste and adjust sweetness if desired.
3. Pour into a glass and enjoy this creamy and nutrient-packed smoothie.

4. Chocolate Coconut Almond Smoothie

<u>*Ingredients*</u>:
- 1 banana, frozen
- 1 tablespoon cocoa powder
- 1/4 cup shredded coconut
- 1 tablespoon almond butter
- 1 cup coconut milk or milk of choice
- Ice cubes (optional)

<u>*Instructions*</u>:
1. Blend frozen banana, cocoa powder, shredded coconut, almond butter, and coconut milk until smooth.
2. Add ice cubes if desired and blend again until creamy.
3. Pour into a glass and indulge in this chocolatey coconut almond delight.

5. Citrus Kale Ginger Smoothie

<u>*Ingredients*</u>:
- 1 cup kale leaves, stems removed
- 1/2 cup frozen mango chunks
- 1/2 inch fresh ginger, peeled
- Juice of 1/2 orange
- 1 tablespoon honey or agave syrup (optional)
- 1 cup water or coconut water

<u>*Instructions*</u>:

1. Blend kale leaves, frozen mango chunks, fresh ginger, orange juice, honey or agave syrup, and water or coconut water until smooth.
2. Adjust sweetness and consistency to your liking.
3. Pour into a glass and enjoy this refreshing citrus kale ginger smoothie.

These customizable smoothie recipes allow you to tailor ingredients and flavors to your preferences while ensuring you get the nutritional benefits you need. Experiment with different combinations to discover your favorite smoothie creations that support your weight loss journey and overall wellness.

Smoothie Challenges and Plans: 7-Day and 30-Day Smoothie Weight Loss Plans, Motivation, and Accountability

Smoothie challenges offer structured plans to help readers incorporate nutritious smoothies into their daily routines for weight loss and overall health. These plans provide motivation and accountability, making it easier to achieve health goals effectively.

Benefits of Smoothie Challenges:

1.Nutrient-Rich: Packed with vitamins, minerals, and antioxidants to support overall health.

2. Convenient: Quick and easy to prepare, ideal for busy lifestyles.

3. Weight Loss Support: Helps manage calorie intake while providing essential nutrients.

4. Variety: Offers a range of flavors and ingredients to keep meals interesting.

7-Day Smoothie Weight Loss Plan

Day 1: Green Detox Smoothie

Ingredients:
- 1 cup spinach
- 1/2 cucumber, peeled and chopped
- 1/2 green apple, chopped
- Juice of 1/2 lemon
- 1 tablespoon chia seeds
- 1 cup coconut water or water

Instructions:
1. Blend spinach, cucumber, green apple, lemon juice, chia seeds, and coconut water until smooth.
2. Pour into a glass and enjoy this refreshing detoxifying smoothie.

Day 2: Berry Blast Smoothie

<u>*Ingredients*</u>:
- 1/2 cup mixed berries (strawberries, blueberries, raspberries)
- 1 banana
- 1/2 cup Greek yogurt
- 1 tablespoon honey (optional)
- 1 cup almond milk or milk of choice

<u>*Instructions*</u>:

1. Blend mixed berries, banana, Greek yogurt, honey, and almond milk until smooth.

2. Pour into a glass and savor this antioxidant-rich smoothie.

Day 3: Tropical Turmeric Smoothie

<u>*Ingredients*</u>:
- 1 cup frozen pineapple chunks
- 1/2 cup frozen mango chunks
- 1/2 inch fresh ginger, peeled
- 1/2 teaspoon ground turmeric
- 1 cup coconut water or water

<u>*Instructions*</u>:

1. Blend pineapple chunks, mango chunks, ginger, turmeric, and coconut water until smooth.

2. Pour into a glass and enjoy this immune-boosting tropical smoothie.

Day 4: Chocolate Avocado Protein Smoothie

Ingredients:
- 1/2 avocado
- 1 scoop chocolate protein powder
- 1 tablespoon almond butter
- 1 tablespoon cocoa powder
- 1 cup almond milk or milk of choice

Instructions:
1. Blend avocado, chocolate protein powder, almond butter, cocoa powder, and almond milk until smooth.
2. Pour into a glass and indulge in this creamy and protein-packed smoothie.

Day 5: Blueberry Kale Smoothie

Ingredients:
- 1 cup kale leaves, stems removed
- 1/2 cup frozen blueberries
- 1/2 banana
- Juice of 1/2 lemon
- 1 tablespoon chia seeds
- 1 cup coconut water or water

Instructions:
1. Blend kale leaves, frozen blueberries, banana, lemon juice, chia seeds, and coconut water until smooth.
2. Pour into a glass and enjoy this refreshing and nutrient-packed smoothie.

30-Day Smoothie Weight Loss Plan

This plan can be repeated weekly with variations to maintain interest and maximize nutritional intake.

Week 1: Detox and Refresh
- Incorporate detoxifying green smoothies and antioxidant-rich berry smoothies.

Week 2: Protein Boost
- Focus on high-protein smoothies with ingredients like Greek yogurt, protein powder, and nut butter.

Week 3: Superfood Power
- Introduce superfoods like chia seeds, flaxseeds, and spirulina into smoothies for added nutrition.

Week 4: Fiber-Rich and Satisfying
- Include fiber-packed smoothies with ingredients such as oats, avocado, and spinach to promote fullness.

Smoothie Challenge Guidelines:

1. Daily Accountability: Encourage participants to track their smoothie intake and share experiences for support.

2. Recipe Variety: Provide a range of recipes to prevent monotony and cater to different tastes.

3. Ingredient Flexibility: Allow substitutions based on dietary preferences and ingredient availability.

Conclusion

Smoothie challenges offer an effective way to jumpstart a healthy lifestyle and achieve weight loss goals with delicious and nutrient-packed smoothies. Encourage readers to customize recipes and adapt plans to fit their individual needs for sustainable results.

These plans and guidelines will help your readers embark on their smoothie journey with structure and motivation, ensuring they enjoy tasty and healthy shakes while achieving their weight loss goals.

Conclusion: Embracing a Healthy Lifestyle with Smoothies

Incorporating smoothies into your daily routine isn't just about enjoying delicious flavors—it's about making a commitment to your health and well-being. Throughout this book, you've discovered the power of smoothies as a tool for weight loss and overall wellness. As we conclude this journey, let's reflect on the long-term benefits and practical tips for maintaining a healthy lifestyle with smoothies.

Long-Term Benefits of Incorporating Smoothies

1. Nutrient-Rich Fuel: Smoothies provide a concentrated source of vitamins, minerals, and antioxidants essential for optimal health.

2. Weight Management: By controlling portion sizes and ingredients, smoothies can support weight loss and weight maintenance goals.

3. Digestive Health: High-fiber ingredients like fruits, vegetables, and seeds promote digestion and gut health.

4. Energy Boost: Nutrient-dense smoothies provide sustained energy levels throughout the day.

5. Hydration: Smoothies made with water, coconut water, or milk contribute to daily hydration needs.

Encouragement and Tips for Maintaining a Healthy Lifestyle

1. Consistency is Key: Incorporate smoothies into your daily routine as a convenient and nutritious meal or snack option.

2. Variety: Experiment with different combinations of fruits, vegetables, proteins, and superfoods to keep your smoothies exciting and nutritious.

3. Balanced Nutrition: Ensure each smoothie contains a balance of proteins, healthy fats, fiber, and carbohydrates to support overall health.

4. Portion Control: Pay attention to portion sizes and avoid overloading smoothies with excess sugars or calorie-dense ingredients.

5. Lifestyle Integration: Use smoothies as part of a holistic approach to wellness, including regular physical activity and adequate sleep.

Final Thoughts

Smoothies offer a flexible and delicious way to support your health journey, whether you're aiming for weight loss, increased energy, or improved overall well-being. By embracing the recipes and guidelines provided in this book, you've equipped yourself with the tools to make informed choices and nourish your body effectively.

Remember, the journey to a healthier lifestyle is unique to each individual. Embrace the journey, celebrate your successes, and continue exploring new ways to enjoy the benefits of smoothies in your everyday life.

Here's to your health, happiness, and the joy of tasty and healthy smoothies!

This conclusion summarizes the key benefits of smoothies and offers practical advice for integrating them into a sustainable and healthy lifestyle. It encourages readers to continue their journey towards wellness with enthusiasm and commitment.

www.ingramcontent.com/pod-product-compliance
Lightning Source LLC
Chambersburg PA
CBHW050822250726

48653CB00006B/2379